Finding the Helpers

Together We Can: Pandemic

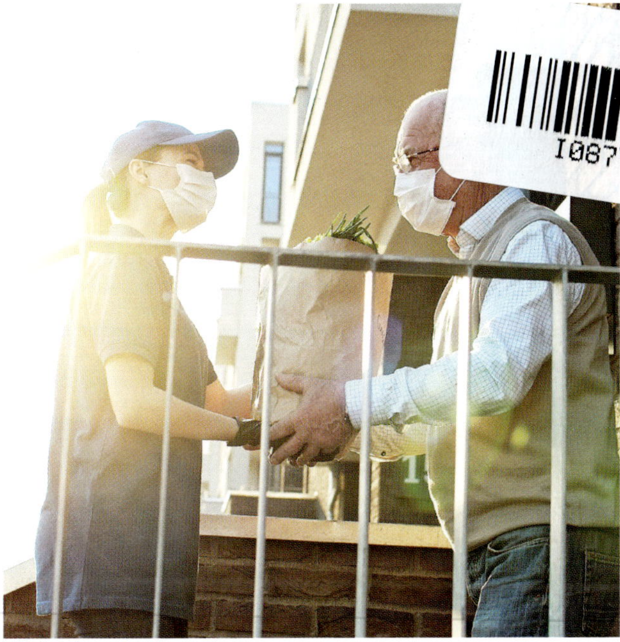

By Shannon Stocker

21st Century Junior Library

CHERRY LAKE PRESS

Published in the United States of America by Cherry Lake Publishing Group
Ann Arbor, Michigan
www.cherrylakepublishing.com

Reading Adviser: Marla Conn, MS, Ed., Literacy specialist, Read-Ability, Inc.

Photo Credits: © VesnaArt/Shutterstock.com, cover, 1; © JessicaGirvan/Shutterstock.com, 4; © Tayvay/Shutterstock.com, 6; © VatsalSheth/Shutterstock.com, 8; © MikeDotta/Shutterstock.com, 10; © Andrew Angelov/Shutterstock.com, 12; © Maria Wan/Shutterstock.com, 14; © Hananeko_Studio/Shutterstock.com, 16; © Veja/Shutterstock.com, 18; © Tada Images/Shutterstock.com, 20

Cherry Lake Press is an imprint of Cherry Lake Publishing Group.

Library of Congress Cataloging-in-Publication Data

Names: Stocker, Shannon, author.
Title: Finding the helpers / Shannon Stocker.
Description: Ann Arbor : Cherry Lake Publishing, 2021. | Series: Together we can: pandemic | Includes index. | Audience: Grades 2-3 | Summary: "The COVID-19 pandemic introduced many changes into children's lives. Finding the Helpers recognizes the heroes kids encounter every day, who are taking risks and spending time to be sure we all have the necessities. This book gives actionable suggestions to help young readers locate the helpers in their own lives in order to get the support they need. Includes science content, based on current CDC recommendations, as well as social emotional content to help with personal wellness and development of empathy. All books in the 21st Century Junior Library encourage readers to think critically and creatively, and use their problem-solving skills. Book includes table of contents, sidebars, glossary, index, and author biography"—Provided by publisher.
Identifiers: LCCN 2020039969 (print) | LCCN 2020039970 (ebook) | ISBN 9781534180147 (hardcover) | ISBN 9781534181854 (paperback) | ISBN 9781534181151 (pdf) | ISBN 9781534182868 (ebook)
Subjects: LCSH: COVID-19 (Disease)—Social aspects—Juvenile literature. | Epidemics—Social aspects—Juvenile literature. | Medical personnel—Juvenile literature. | Community life—Juvenile literature. | Heroes—Juvenile literature.
Classification: LCC RA644.C67 S746 2021 (print) | LCC RA644.C67 (ebook) | DDC 362.1962/414—dc23
LC record available at https://lccn.loc.gov/2020039969
LC ebook record available at https://lccn.loc.gov/2020039970

Cherry Lake Publishing Group would like to acknowledge the work of the Partnership for 21st Century Learning, a Network of Battelle for Kids. Please visit http://www.battelleforkids.org/networks/p21 for more information.

Printed in the United States of America
Corporate Graphics

CONTENTS

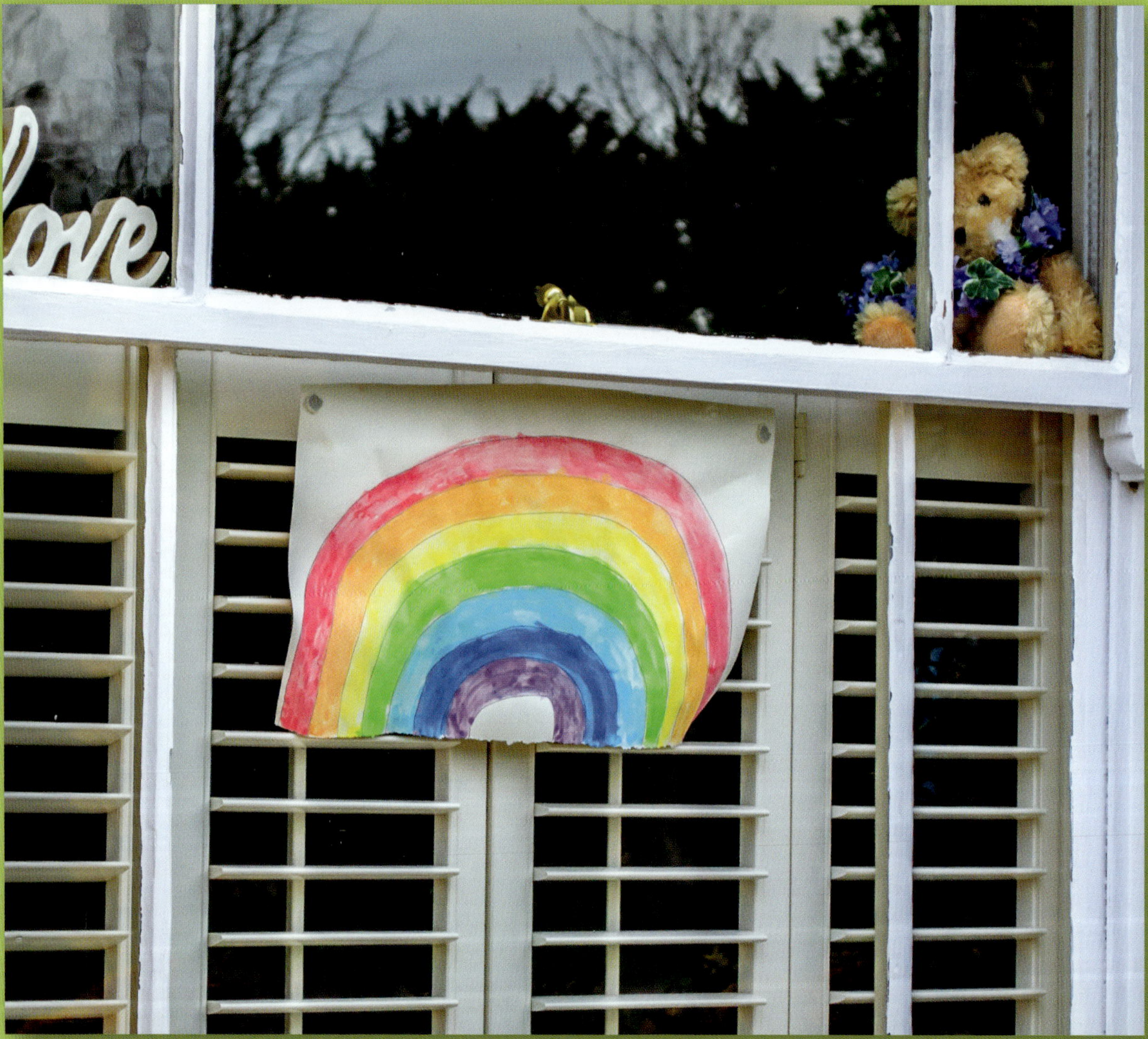

How many rainbows in windows do you see in your neighborhood?

Healing Helpers

Have you ever noticed all the people around you who do good things for others? There are lots of them! And guess what? You don't have to be a grown-up to help others. You can be a helper too.

During a **pandemic**, people who help others are like rainbows. They give us hope and make us happy, even on rainy days. That's why some families put rainbows in their windows. They're helping to add a little sunshine to their communities.

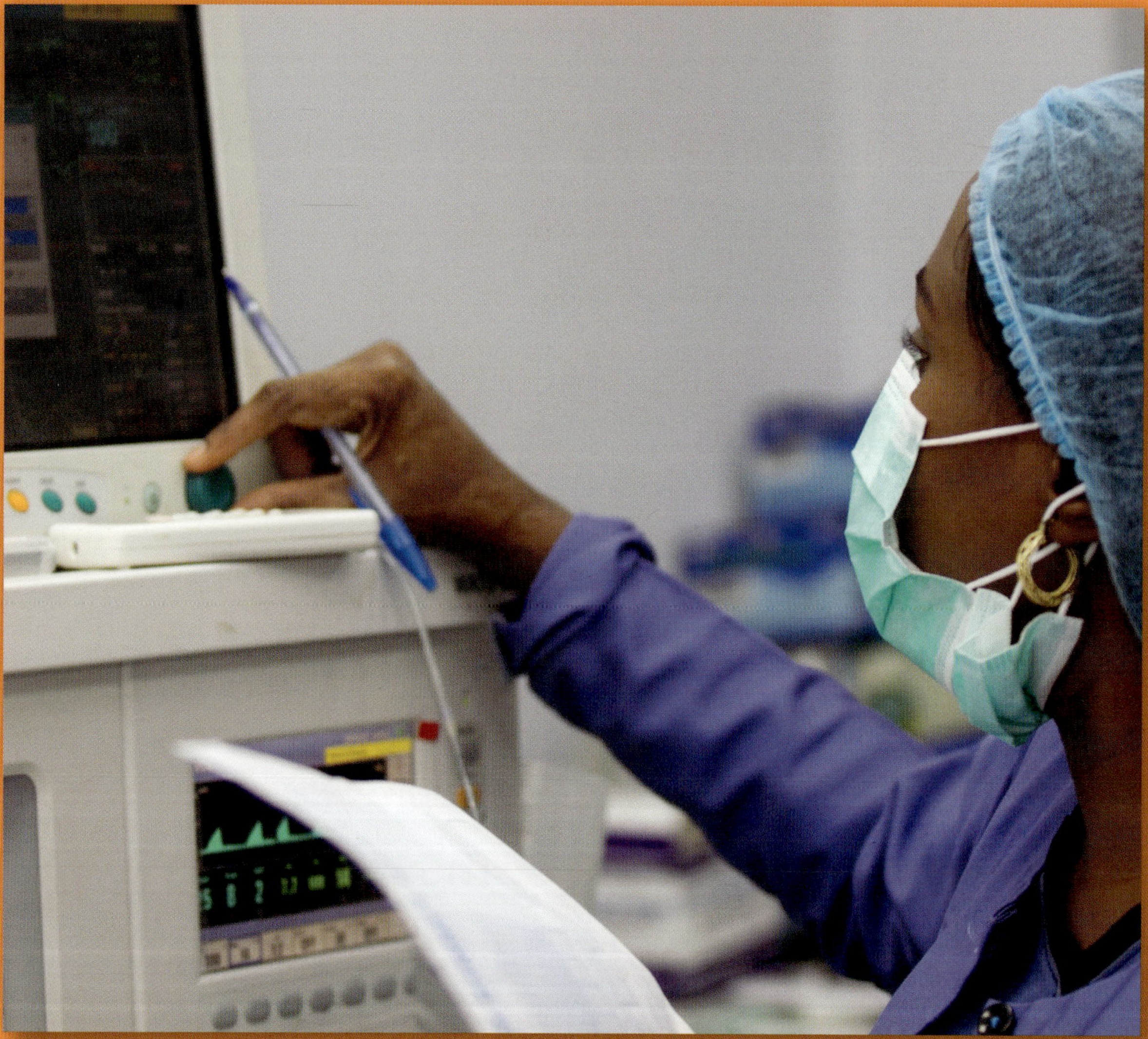

Around the world, doctors work hard to control the coronavirus.

Doctors, nurses, dentists, and other healthcare workers have risked their lives every day during the **coronavirus** pandemic. They are called **essential workers** because they are needed to keep our communities running. But they make sacrifices too. At home, they have to keep their loved ones safe. These workers often live in a different part of their house so they don't **infect** family members. They work many hours, and they risk their lives every single day. They are very important healing helpers.

Think!

How many different types of healthcare providers can you name?

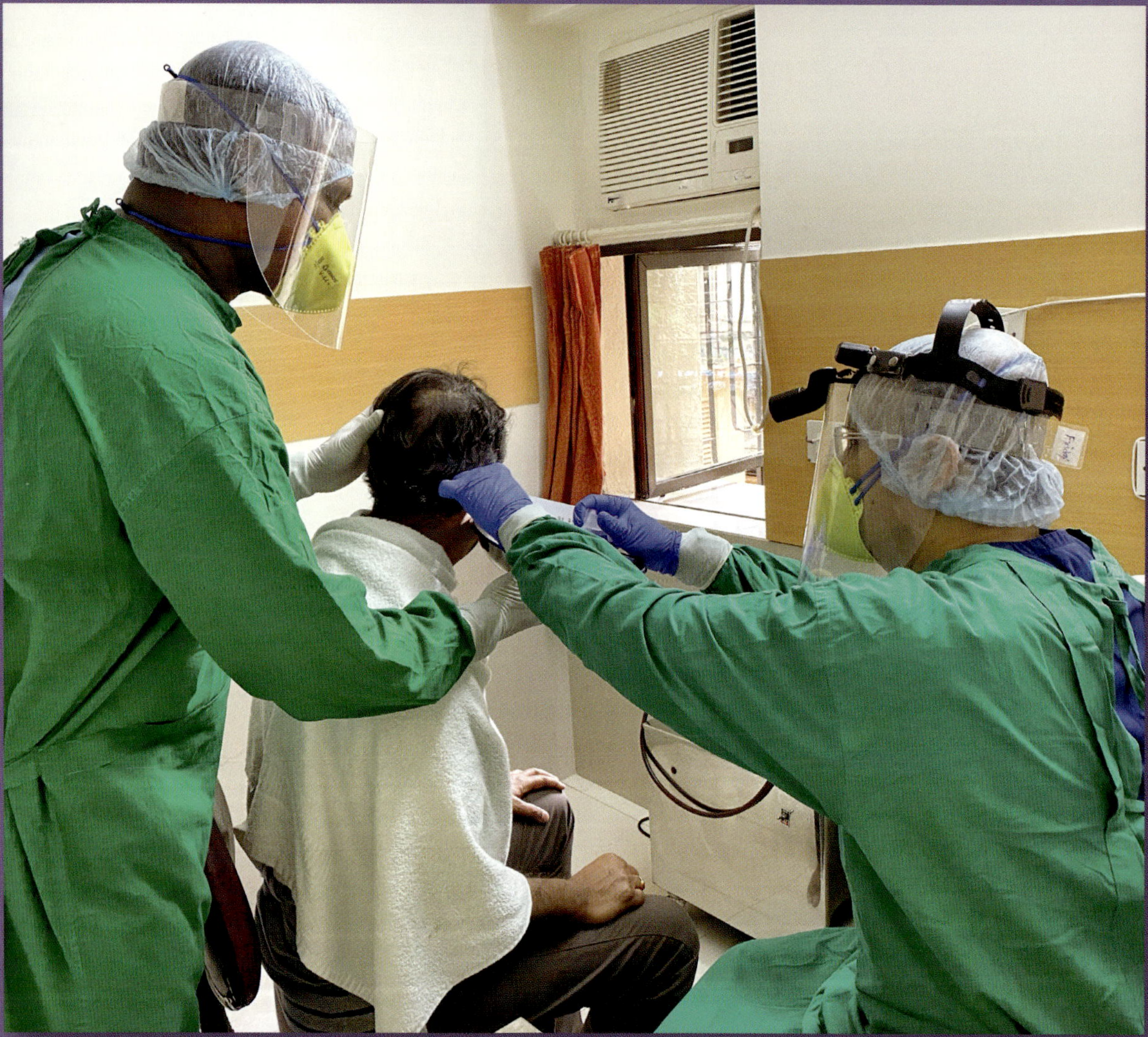

Special clothing and equipment—called personal protective equipment (PPE)—keep our healthcare workers safe and healthy.

When your doctor prescribes a medication, **pharmacists** make sure you get the correct kind and **dosage**. They are essential workers too. People often call their pharmacists with questions about the virus and how to get a **COVID-19** test. They also call if they are worried about not having enough medication or not being able to get it on time. Many pharmacies have been delivering medications for free, to limit the number of people coming into the store.

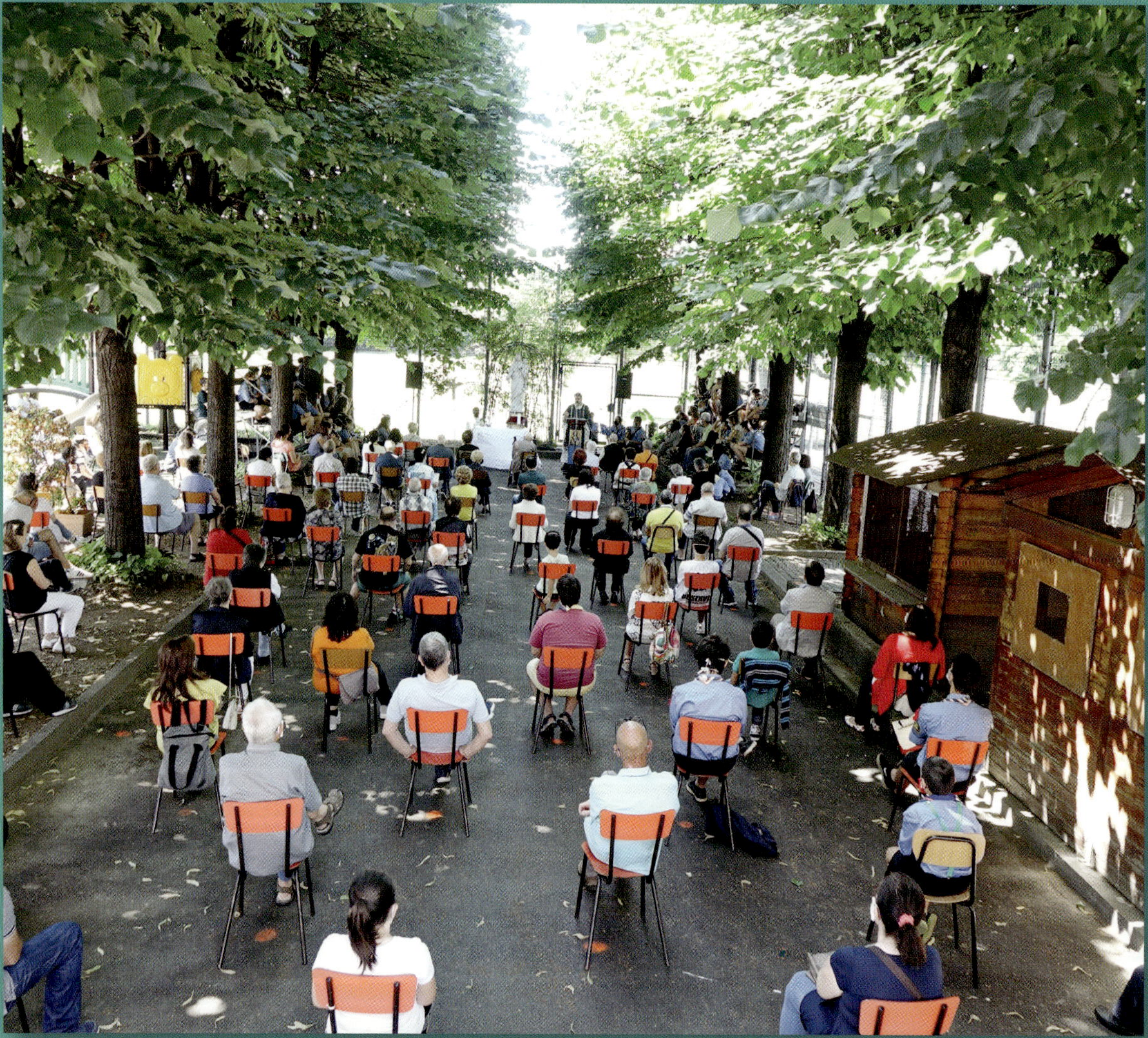

Some places of worship also offer services outside.

Religious leaders are healing helpers too. A pandemic can make many people feel lonely and sad, especially during holidays that are usually celebrated with family and friends. Many religious leaders have offered ways to worship **virtually**. They also make themselves available for the sick and needy. They help keep our hearts and spirits healthy.

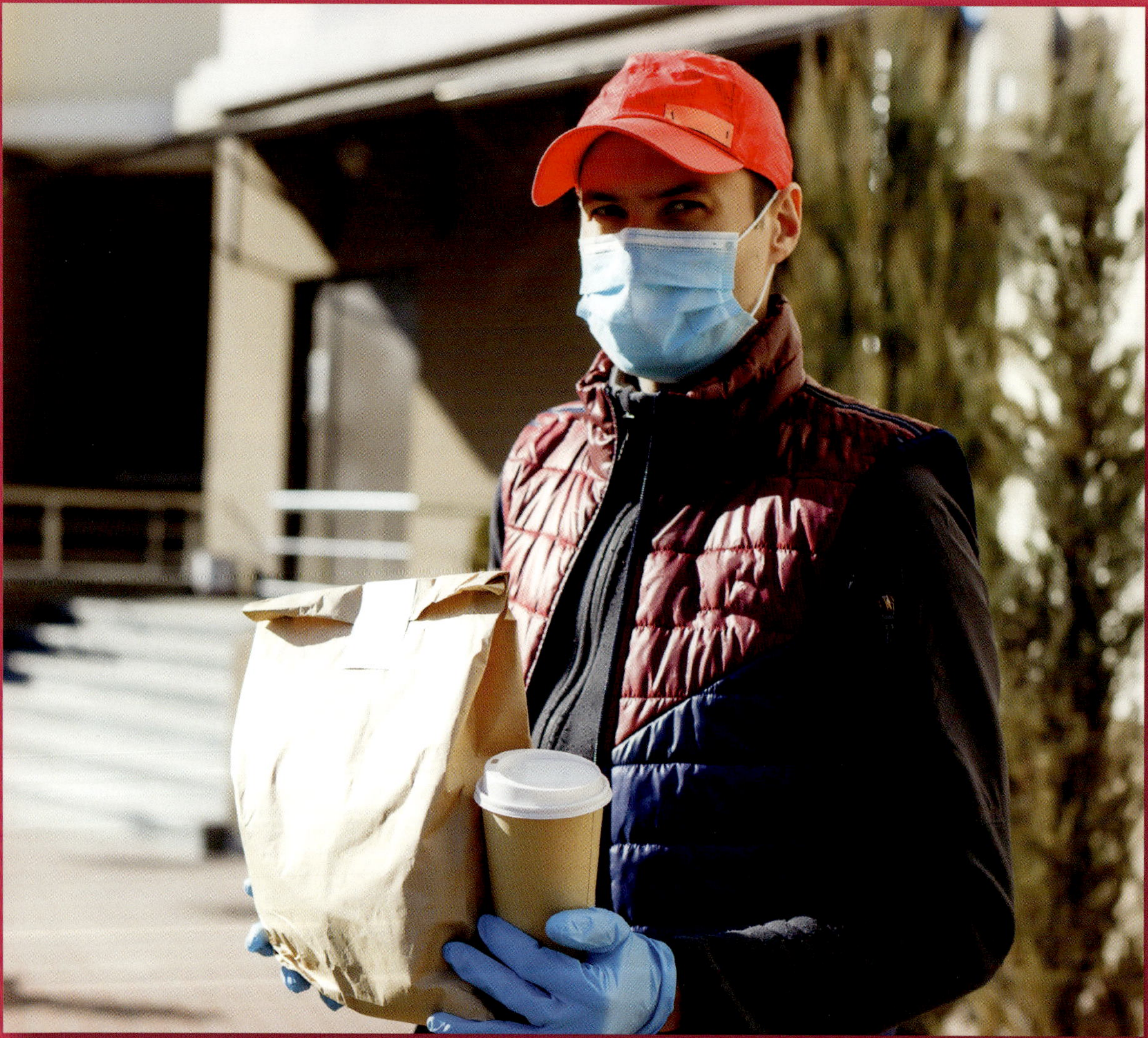

Delivery workers are taking a risk—thank them by wearing a mask when you answer the door!

Community Helpers

Lots of people recognize healing helpers as essential workers. But there are many **unsung heroes** in our communities too. Delivery workers bring us groceries, packages, school supplies, prepared food, mail, and more. Almost anything you need can be delivered straight to your door during a pandemic.

Think!

In 1914, 4-year-old Charlotte May Pierstorff's parents mailed her to her grandparents by train. What is the weirdest thing you've sent by mail?

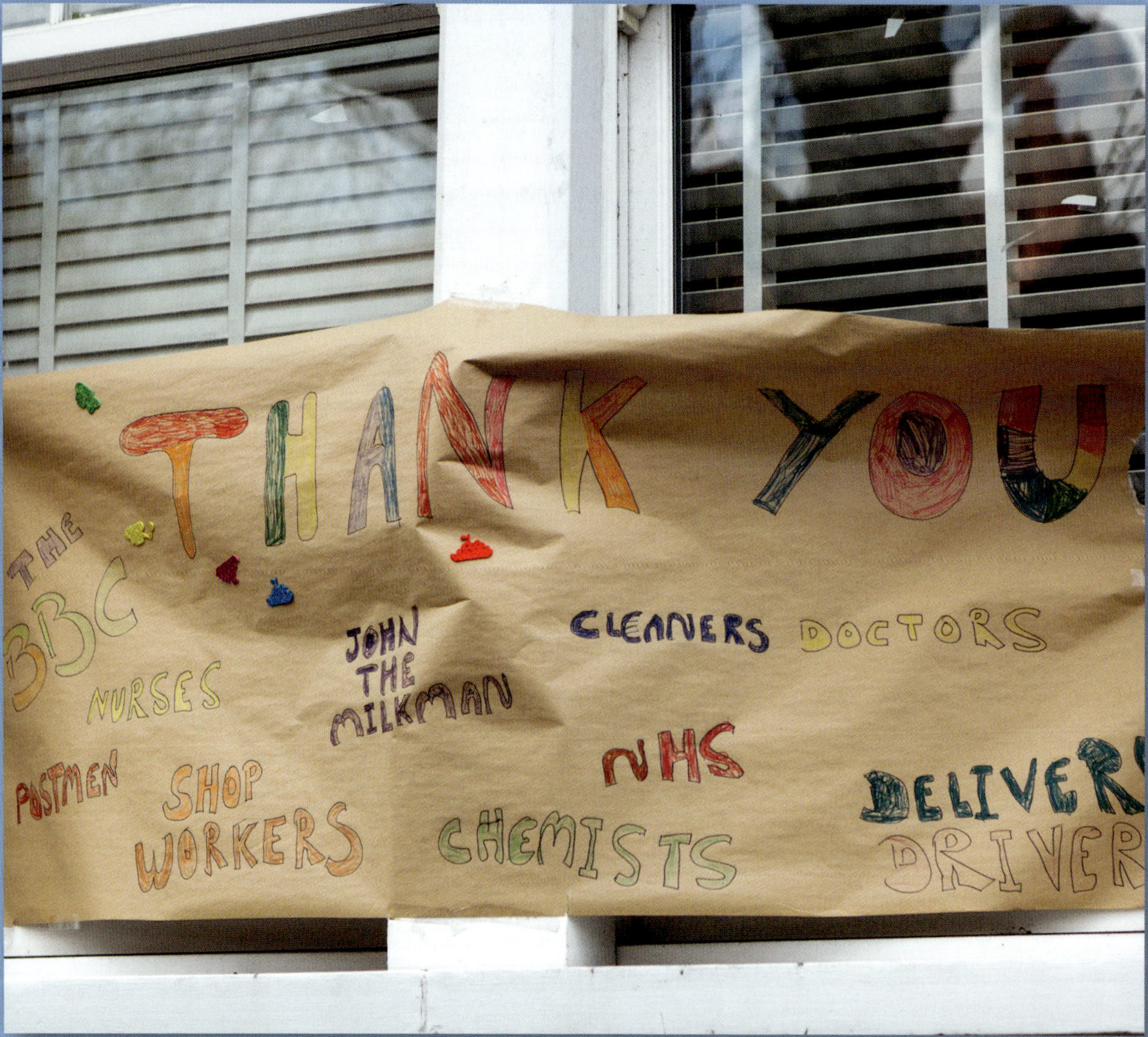
THANK YOU
THE BBC
NURSES
JOHN THE MILKMAN
CLEANERS
DOCTORS
POSTMEN
SHOP WORKERS
NHS
CHEMISTS
DELIVERY DRIVER

You can thank community helpers by making signs or drawing pictures for them.

It takes a lot of helpers to make a community function. We need grocery store workers, sanitation workers, plumbers, soldiers, electricians, bus drivers, firefighters, farmers, postal service workers, and many others. All of these people have jobs that are essential for keeping our communities and homes running smoothly.

Think!

Can you name another job that's essential?

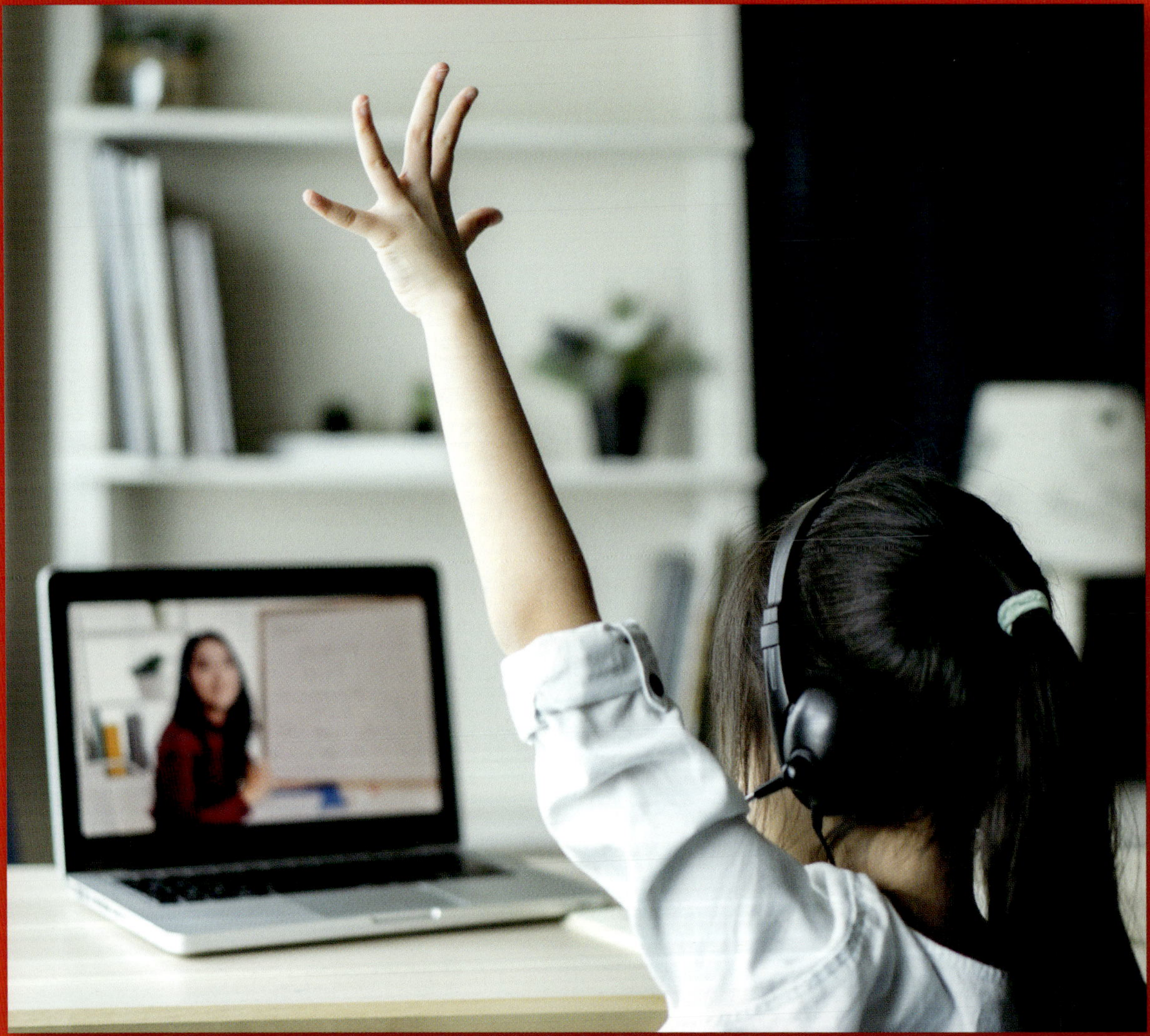

What are some ways online school is hard for you?
How do you think it is hard for teachers?

Helpers at Home

During the school year, who helps you learn—even when you're stuck at home? Teachers! They have one of the most important jobs in our society because they shape the world's future leaders (like you!). They do more than just teach math, writing, and other subjects. They help provide structure so you learn how to manage your time. They guide you through friendships and arguments with classmates. They encourage you to be the best you can be.

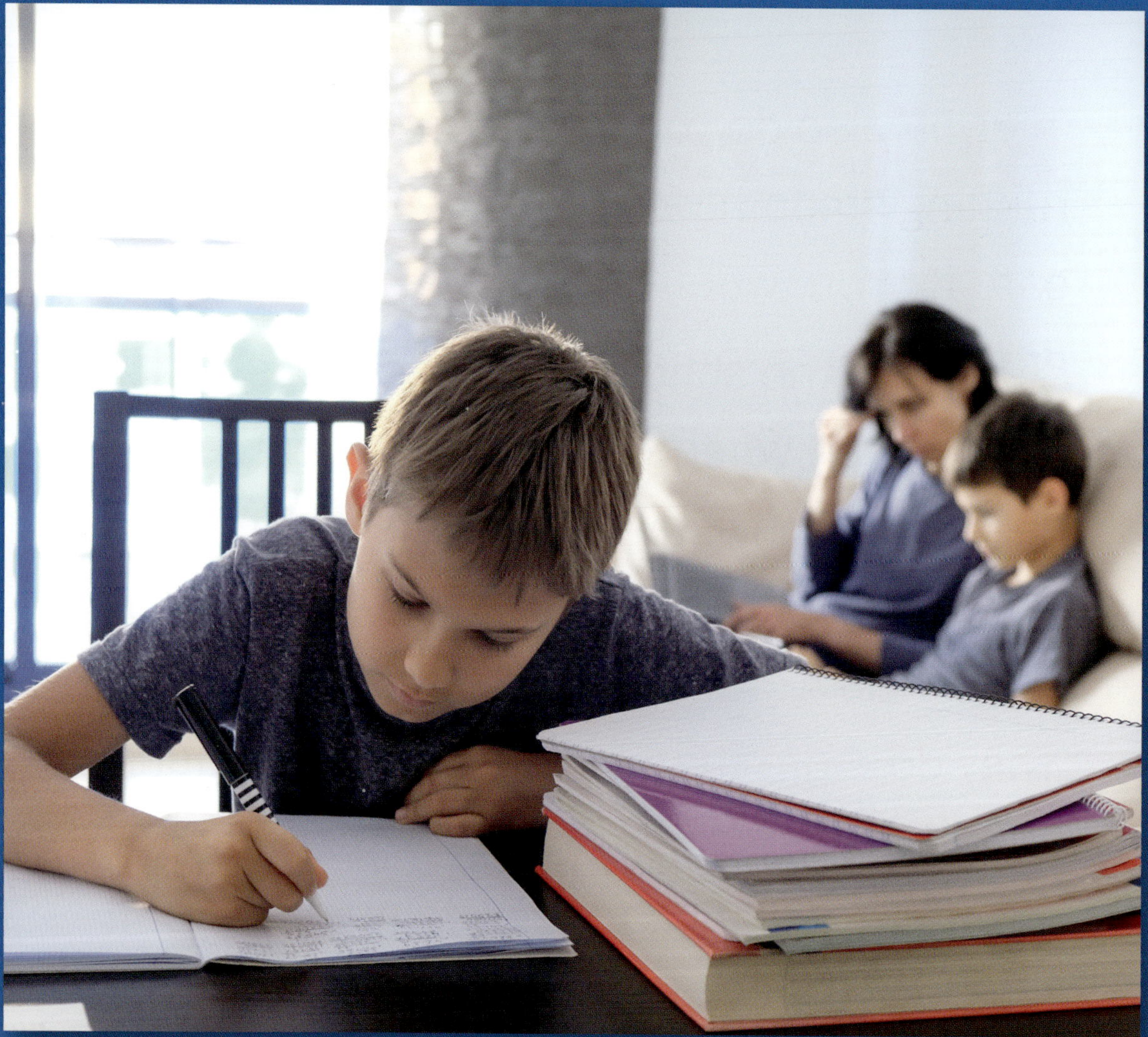

You can be a helper at home by doing your homework when asked.

Who else do you think keeps your home running smoothly? The grown-ups who care for you, whether they are your parents, grandparents, or other adults. They are responsible for keeping you fed, dressed, and healthy. That can be a lot of work, but you make it all worthwhile!

Create!

A homemade card can make a grown-up feel loved and appreciated.

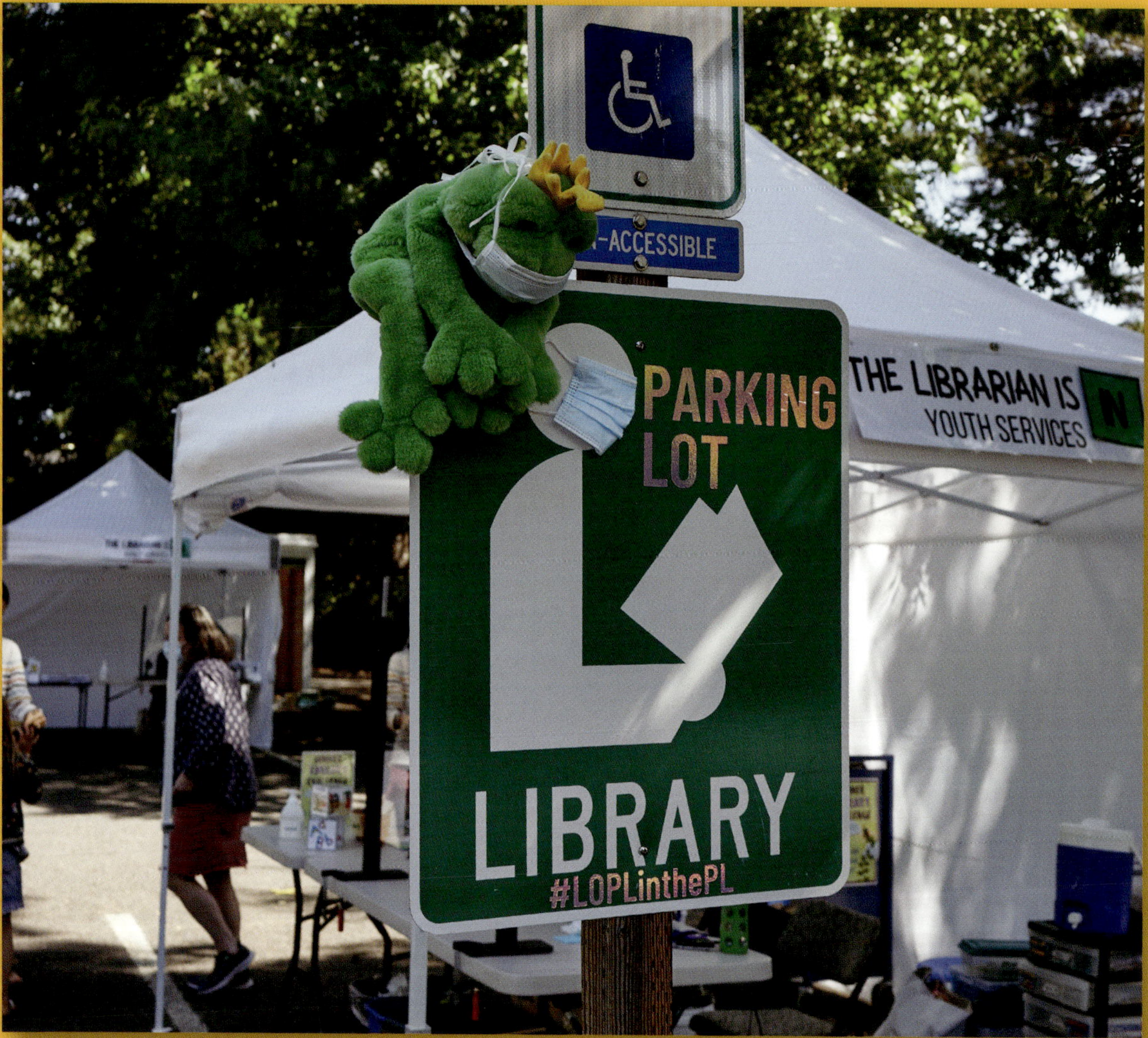

Librarians work hard so you can bring books home, even during a pandemic.

Did you know that some of the most important jobs during a pandemic are the ones that YOU can do? You can keep essential workers healthy by staying home and washing your hands frequently. If you have to go out, wear a cloth mask and practice **social distancing** to keep others safe. Whatever the job, all essential workers can be called by the same name—hero!

GLOSSARY

coronavirus (kuh-ROH-nuh-vye-ruhs) a family of viruses that cause a variety of illnesses in people and other mammals

COVID-19 (KOH-vid nine-TEEN) the name of the disease caused by the coronavirus

dosage (DOHS-ij) the amount of medicine a person should take

essential workers (ih-SEN-shuhl WUR-kurz) people who provide work that's necessary to keep a community safe and healthy

infect (in-FEKT) to cause disease by introducing germs or viruses

pandemic (pan-DEM-ik) an outbreak of a disease that affects a large part of the population

pharmacists (FAHR-muh-sists) people trained to prepare and give out drugs and medicines

social distancing (SOH-shuhl DIS-tuhns-ing) the act of staying at least 6 feet (2 meters) away from others

unsung heroes (UHN-suhng HEER-ohz) people who do great deeds or have committed acts of bravery, but are not recognized

virtually (VUR-choo-uhl-ee) accessed by a computer, especially online

FIND OUT MORE

WEBSITES

CDC—Talking with Children about Coronavirus Disease 2019
https://www.cdc.gov/coronavirus/2019-ncov/daily-life-coping/talking-with-children.html

Education.com—Lesson Plan: Helpers in Our Community
https://www.education.com/lesson-plan/helpers-in-our-community

ESL/EFL Preschool Teachers—Community Helpers Worksheets and More
https://eflpreschoolteachers.blogspot.com/2016/05/community-helpers-worksheets-and-more.html

Massachusetts General Hospital—Family Values-Based Communication: How Parents Can Talk with Their Children about Their Roles When They Are Essential Workers
https://www.massgeneral.org/children/coronavirus/how-parents-can-talk-with-children-about-roles-as-essential-workers

Totschooling—Community Helpers Printable Paper Hats
https://www.totschooling.net/2017/08/community-helpers-printable-paper-hats.html?m=1

INDEX

ABOUT THE AUTHOR

Shannon Stocker writes picture books, books for young readers, and *Chicken Soup* stories. Her family likes to thank helpers by leaving notes of gratitude in sidewalk chalk and putting hearts and rainbows in their windows. Shannon lives in Louisville, Kentucky, with Greg, Cassidy, Tye, and far too many critters.